T L BROOKS

Silence

This book was professionally typeset on Reedsy.
Find out more at reedsy.com

Contents

1	Chapter 1	1
2	Chapter 2	6
3	Chapter 3	8
4	Chapter 4	12
5	Chapter 5	15
6	Chapter 6	17
7	Chapter 7	20
8	Chapter 8	27
9	Chapter 9	29
10	Chapter 10	31
11	Chapter 11	34
12	REFERENCES	36

1

Chapter 1

This day began like any other day for us. It was late morning; we grabbed our coffee, jumped in our truck, and headed to the city from our rural town for my dentist appointment. It was a beautiful, crisp morning in early January of the year 2023. I enjoyed the gorgeous countryside as we traveled along the highway. Watching the pastures of cows and horses eating grass without a care in the world was so peaceful. Now and again, I would get a glimpse of deer forging on fields of flowers and grass in the distance. I loved the drive. I hadn't had my teeth cleaned by a dentist in a few years, so I was excited to go. Weird, I know! My husband thinks so, too! As a child, I went to the dentist regularly, so I have never feared the dentist. Also, the dentist I had been going to for the last couple of decades happened to be the sister of a friend of mine from childhood.

As I sit in this new, strange dentist's office waiting room, waiting to be called back, my mind wanders to what my husband and I have been doing over the last several years to prepare for our move. We made several trips to Texas, together and apart, helped two of our adult children and their families move here, dropped our youngest off at college, and then returned to Southern California and finished preparing our house to sell.

It has been an exhausting three years, but we finally made it!

When I say "prepare" our house, I am not talking about just paint and a few "staging" items; I am talking about almost a complete renovation inside and out! When we bought the house over seventeen years ago, we had every intention of renovating it immediately, but life kept getting in the way. I am sure you can relate! The only room that we completely remodeled shortly after purchase was the kitchen because, for a family of six, it didn't work for us. There was no pantry, and the doorway was so small our refrigerator didn't fit through it!

When we were house hunting, the kids and I loved the house, but my husband was not so fond of it because it was a project. Even though it needed A LOT of work, he knew we needed it because we were a family of six living in a very small two-bedroom, one-bath house. We have three daughters and one son, and our son needed a room of his own. The home was built in the 1950s. It had a sunken living room, an old brick fireplace, and a huge picture window with a beautiful view of the snow-capped mountains. Sitting above the living room was a good-sized dining area next to the kitchen, and down the hall were two bedrooms, a bathroom in the hall, an office with a bathroom, and the master suite, which had a small bathroom and a small room off to the side. The home was almost 2000 square feet. It sat on nearly an acre, atop a small hill with privacy from the street and the neighbors; it had a large built-in pool and plenty of room for the kids to play outside. SOLD!

We all moved into the master suite temporarily because all the rooms required new flooring and paint before the children could move into them. The children picked their rooms; our oldest daughter and our son would have their own rooms, and the youngest two daughters would share. (Our son was wise; he took the room with its bathroom. He knew he didn't want to share with three girls anymore!) We first completed the oldest children's rooms and then moved on to the room our two younger daughters would share. Their room would require additional time as we needed to close off a wall and doorway, install a new door opposite the bathroom, and construct a closet.

We moved to the kitchen remodel once the children's bedrooms were complete. We completely stripped it back to the studs and upgraded the electrical to accommodate new appliances, removed the sitting area for two, made it a large walk-in pantry, and widened the doorway to the dining area. The kitchen was complete with new insulation, drywall, a dual pane window, cabinets, appliances, paint, fixtures, and flooring! Once we completed the kitchen, life got busy (for years), and the rest of the house pretty much stayed the same.

Since life got busy for over seventeen years, we had a HUGE renovation project! But we were determined to get it done, move to Texas, and start anew. In the beginning, we had the help of family, but within a year, they all moved to Texas, and then it was only us. We often became overwhelmed as we jumped from one project to another. It seemed like we were not finishing any of the projects, prompting us to adopt a more organized approach.

As needed, we demolished, repaired, and remodeled room-by-room, from the ceiling to the floor. We only hired some contractors for big jobs that we could not do. We hired one for the roof and another for the stucco, and we completed the rest ourselves with the help of one friend. Seven days a week, fourteen-to-sixteen-hour days, over five hundred days, through Covid-19, material delays, and shutdowns, our house was ready for the market! SOLD!

"Tammy." I look up and see a dentist assistant smile at me, holding the door open. I get up and follow her back. She takes me to a room in the back and has me sit in the dental chair. She put the "bib" on me and asked me all the usual questions for a new patient. She then asked me if it was okay to take my blood pressure. I have been going to the dentist my whole life and never had them take my blood pressure. I wondered if this was a new thing or a Texas thing. I had no reservations about her taking my blood pressure since I have always had low to normal blood pressure. In fact, most automatic machines had difficulty reading my blood pressure. My average blood pressure reading would be 90/60 to 110/65.

She proceeds to put on the blood pressure cuff and take my blood pressure. She takes one reading and writes down the numbers. She retakes it. Taking the stethoscope out of her ears, she asks, "Do you take blood pressure medicine?"

"No, why?" I ask.

"Because your blood pressure is extremely high. It is 171/106," says the dental assistant. I am surprised, and my mind starts racing. I don't understand. How can my blood pressure be so high? Why?

"Are you nervous about coming to the dentist?" she asked.

"No," I respond.

"Sometimes your blood pressure can increase if you are anxious or nervous about something," she explains. I know that I am not nervous about getting my teeth cleaned, so that's not the reason. At this point, I am just confused and don't understand why my blood pressure would be so high.

"I am sorry, but we cannot clean your teeth until you see your doctor. It is unsafe for us to clean your teeth with high blood pressure," she explains. I tell her I understand and leave the room.

I went outside, and my husband looked at me and said, "That was fast!" I got in the truck, and he followed.

"They couldn't clean my teeth," I said.

"Why not?" he asks cautiously.

"Because my blood pressure was 171/106!" I said as my voice cracks and tears are forming in my eyes.

We have been married for over thirty-five years, and he knows me well. He will not press me, especially when I am on the verge of tears. He knows that I will talk to him when I am ready.

"I will text my doctor when we get home and make an appointment for you," he says quietly. I nod. I am quiet for the ride home.

2

Chapter 2

Some of you may be wondering why I would get so emotional over high blood pressure. I asked myself the same question that day and several weeks after that. Even today, I am not sure if I know the answer to that question (for sure), but here are my thoughts.

It is not that I was unfamiliar with high blood pressure; it runs in my husband's family. His mother, sister, and brother have all taken blood pressure medicine for as long as I can remember. Except for them having high blood pressure and taking medicine for it, I didn't have much knowledge beyond this. Just recently, my husband also had to be put on high blood pressure medicine. He had high blood pressure for a long time but refused to admit it and, therefore, never took medicine for it. He is a stubborn one!

He was lucky that his high blood pressure presented in the way that it did and not a stroke or heart attack. It started as a light nosebleed that gradually worsened and continued over a couple of days. He had not had a nosebleed in decades, so it "freaked" him out! Unfortunately, I was on one of the trips to Texas and could not take him into urgent care, so our son had to take him. They took his blood pressure, and it was through the roof (*a lot* higher than my reading)!

Since the doctor prescribed my husband medication for high blood pressure, I learned a little more about it, but nothing beyond what the doctor told us. I guess you could say I had the attitude that it was his family that had the history, so I only needed to know what the doctor told us.

My husband could have better habits, eating or otherwise. He smokes, drinks, and loves to snack. He loves chips but especially LOVES eating a whole, large pepperoni Digiorno's pizza or twenty chicken nuggets and French fries as a midnight snack! He eats this almost every night. (He is not overweight.) I have always told him, "If I ate like you, I would weigh 500 pounds!!!" We laugh.

Even after my husband was diagnosed with high blood pressure and began taking his prescribed medication, he hasn't changed his habits. I could nag him to make changes, but I chose not to. I believe each person's life is theirs to live the way they want. Tomorrow is not guaranteed. I love him the way he is, and if he is happy, I am happy.

So, when the dental assistant told me I had high blood pressure that day, it was like a punch in my gut! At some point, I expected my husband to be prescribed medication for high blood pressure because of his family history and bad habits. I **NEVER** expected to be told that I had high blood pressure!

I felt like I had good habits. I rarely drink alcohol. I don't smoke. I seldom eat sweets or desserts; my favorite drinks are unsweetened tea and milk. We rarely eat out. I don't eat junk food all day long, and I don't eat horrible midnight snacks! I typically have oatmeal, bagels, or occasionally eggs and bacon about once a week. My lunches would be sandwiches with fruit, carrots, or celery and an occasional small bag of chips. Our dinners would consist of meat, a vegetable, rice or potatoes, and an occasional salad. Therefore, in my mind, I felt like I ate healthy food and couldn't wrap my head around why I would have high blood pressure. It was very deflating!

3

Chapter 3

My husband contacted his doctor and made an appointment for me the following week. Since we had only recently relocated to Texas and I hadn't established a doctor for myself yet, I didn't mind seeing the same doctor he did. She was friendly, and I liked her. As my appointment approached, we celebrated my 55th birthday with our children and granddaughter over the weekend, which provided a welcome distraction. However, my husband sensed it was bothering me and would attempt to reassure me, suggesting that it was just a "fluke" and everything would turn out fine. Despite his efforts, I still had my doubts.

A couple of days before my appointment, I filled out all the forms online and submitted them so that when I arrived, they could take me right in. For the first time, I was anxious to go to the doctor.

We arrived on the day of my appointment, and my husband asked if I wanted him to accompany me inside. I decided to go in by myself. Once inside, they took me to a room, weighed me, measured my height, and placed me in another room. Shortly after, the nurse returned to check my blood pressure and pulse. After taking them several times, she reassured me everything was okay, and the doctor would be with me shortly, and she left the room.

"Hello Tammy! I am Dr. Nguyen. How are you?" she asks. Dr. Nguyen is of Asian descent and approximately five feet tall. She has a petite frame and sleek black hair. Her striking, large, and captivating green eyes accentuate her delicate face.

"Nervous!" I exclaim.

"Aah, you don't need to be nervous. We will take care of you!" she says kindly. "Your blood pressure is still extremely high, 173/102." My heart sinks. She explains the urgency of starting medication immediately to lower it. Reassuring me, she is confident and pledges to find the underlying cause of this sudden elevation, given my previous history. Sensing my hesitation and distress, she spends considerable time delving into my history, eating habits, exercise, stress levels, and anything else that may be beneficial for her to know. Concerned about the medication, I inquired about its long-term necessity, potential side effects, and the consequences of refusal. Patiently, she addresses all my concerns. We agree that I'll return for a comprehensive fasting blood panel in a week, followed by a review of the results in four weeks. Meanwhile, I consent to the blood pressure medication and pledge to report any side effects.

The week went by quickly, and I returned for the blood test as scheduled.

Over the following four weeks, life continued with its usual busyness, which proved a welcome distraction from my concerns. Adhering to the prescribed medication regimen, I encountered no side effects. However, as the appointment approached, I noticed my anxiety mounting. While part of me yearned to uncover the results, another part hesitated. What if the news wasn't favorable?

I sit here with tears streaming down my face, looking at the results. Everything is in the **RED,** not just slightly red, but ***way over in the red zone***! I don't understand!! I had a physical and a complete blood panel done just a little over two years ago for a life insurance policy, and everything was normal! How did my numbers go from normal to red *so fast* with no changes in my lifestyle? What makes it even harder to hear is just a few months prior, she told my husband that his blood results all came back in the **normal** range! What the HELL!!!

"Tammy, you have the three silent but deadly killers! High blood pressure, high cholesterol, and high A1C! You are not just slightly in the red in these areas. You are on the extreme other end! You are fortunate that you have not had a heart attack or a stroke already." she explained gently but firmly.

My test Results.

Title	Normal Ranges	My Number
A1C	5 – 5.7	11.2
Triglycerides	<150	451
LDL Cholesterol	<130	Unable to read due to Triglycerides over 400

She went on to elaborate on the remaining test results. Not only did the numbers above elevate into the red zone, but my RBC (red blood count), HGB (hemoglobin), and HCT (hematocrit) were also in the red zone, and they found I was deficient in Vitamin D. She clarified the test results also showed I was in the postmenopausal phase, which was taking a toll on my system. She speculated that this hormonal transition might cause sudden and significant changes in my numbers. She also mentioned that my blood had thickened and specific processes were not functioning as they should be.

"I need to put you on medicine for the A1C and the cholesterol."

"Is medication my only alternative? If I start taking medications, will I ever be able to stop? I struggled to come to terms with the idea of relying on medication indefinitely. I'm aware that doctors often prescribe medicines without considering discontinuation. Additionally, I'm sensitive to medication and am apprehensive about the potential for increased dosages and side effects. However, I acknowledge the heightened risk of stroke or heart attack. I felt overwhelmed with frustration and at a loss.

Recognizing my high levels of stress and overwhelm, she extended our conversation. We reached an agreement: I would commence with a low dosage of Metformin, postpone the cholesterol medication, and maintain my blood pressure medication regimen. I committed to monitoring my blood pressure daily and recording the readings for my upcoming doctor's appointment in four weeks. With my prescriptions in hand, I departed.

During my drive, I tried to recall any symptoms or indications from the past few years that may have indicated a problem. However, I couldn't remember experiencing any. I had been feeling well while working on the house and have felt even better since we arrived in Texas. Apart from a few colds over the past few years, I haven't experienced any illnesses.

4

Chapter 4

Blood is forced through your vessels consistently at too high a rate, going undiscovered for a long time—symptomless or symptoms camouflaging themselves as something else, all while causing damage. Sssshhhh, I am a silent but deadly killer! Most don't know I am even causing damage because my symptoms, if any, are mistaken for other very common symptoms. I am high blood pressure, and I can kill you if I go undetected for too long!

There are several studies on high blood pressure; one concluded that 1 in 2 Americans have high blood pressure, and another concluded that 1 in 3 Americans have it. Whichever study is more accurate, that is an alarming number of Americans with high blood pressure! When high blood pressure goes undiscovered for a long time, it can cause many other health problems such as – heart attack or heart failure, stroke, kidney failure or disease, and vision loss; it can weaken the walls of your blood vessels and cause other debilitating diseases. Did you know that someone has a stroke every 40 <u>seconds</u> in the United States? Also, every 3 <u>minutes</u> and 14 seconds in the United States, someone dies from a stroke. I had no idea that some had a stroke or died that often in the

12

United States from issues caused by high blood pressure. I found this information very disturbing!

Remember how I mentioned that my husband was lucky that his high blood pressure presented as a nosebleed? I mentioned that because the American Heart Association stated that evidence has pointed out that high blood pressure does not typically present as nosebleeds. It is *very rare* it will present this way. Other ways it **may** present itself, but they are not considered directly related to high blood pressure: blood spots in the eyes, facial flushing, dizziness, and headaches. The American Heart Association recommends testing your blood pressure if you are experiencing any of these symptoms and feeling unwell. If it is higher than usual, wait five minutes and test it again. If it is still higher than usual, contact your health professional and discuss your symptoms and blood pressure readings.

What do the numbers mean, 120/80? The first number is the systolic pressure. The first number is how much pressure your blood forces against your artery walls when your heart contracts. The second number is the diastolic pressure. The second number is how much pressure your blood forces against your artery walls when your heart rests. Although both numbers are significant, healthcare professionals prioritize the first number, especially those over 50 years. When the first number starts to increase, it could indicate that the arteries are beginning to stiffen or other cardiac issues are arising.

There are five stages of high blood pressure. Normal is when you have regular blood pressure readings of 120/80 or less. Healthcare profession-als consider you to have healthy eating and exercise habits. Elevated is when you have regular blood pressure readings of 120-129/less than 80. Healthcare professionals say you will likely develop high blood pressure in the future if you don't make changes. Hypertension Stage 1 is when you have regular readings of 130-139/80-89. Healthcare professionals say you need to make lifestyle changes now, and they may prescribe high blood pressure medications. You now may be at risk for a heart attack, stroke, or other issues. Hypertension Stage 2 is when you have regular readings of 140/90 or higher. Healthcare professionals will put you on one or a combination of medications and recommend an exercise regimen and a new diet. Hypertensive Crisis is when your blood pressure reading is 180/120; wait five minutes and test your blood pressure again. Contact your healthcare professional immediately if it is still the same or higher. If it is that high and you are experiencing other symptoms such as shortness of breath, back pain, chest pain, or slurred speech, don't wait! Call 9-1-1!

Now that I have given you some basic information on high blood pressure and possible symptoms let me give you some good information. If you have already been diagnosed with high blood pressure, do not be discouraged; you can change your future! You can lessen your chances of, or prevent, a stroke, and you can reduce the amount of medicine you are on or get off it completely. You can prevent a stroke from happening if you become proactive in your health! You must be committed and make some changes in your life! Change your diet, start a regular exercise program, quit smoking, quit drinking (or cut back), and reduce stress.

5

Chapter 5

Aslow plaque buildup along your artery walls decreases the pathway and causes damage while not signaling that danger is in your future. I will make your heart work harder to keep you alive, and I can wreak havoc on your world, and you will not even know I exist! Silently, I wait! I am high cholesterol, and I can squeeze the life out of you!

There is "good" cholesterol and "bad" cholesterol. HDL is good cholesterol, and LDL is bad cholesterol. You need good cholesterol in your system because it has the job of removing the bad cholesterol. The HDL collects (or attaches to) the LDL and takes it to the liver, where it is broken down and expelled. If there is insufficient HDL, the bad cholesterol, LDL, travels through your system and builds up in your arteries, causing plaque that narrows your artery walls. As the artery walls narrow, your heart must pump harder to deliver enough oxygenated blood through your arteries to sustain your system. In turn, this causes your heart to work too hard and, over time, can cause a heart attack or damage to your heart!

Cholesterol is naturally made in our system, and we also get it from certain foods. One-third of our cholesterol profile is from our diet, biosynthesis produced by our liver makes the other third of cholesterol, and the final third is reabsorption into our system. Therefore, we have no control over two-thirds of the cholesterol role within our bodies. With that said, the third we do have control over is diet, which can play a **significant** role in keeping our cholesterol low and **reducing** high cholesterol if we eat healthy.

High blood pressure and high cholesterol can be diagnosed together, as it was with me, but studies have found that high blood pressure does not cause high cholesterol. On the other hand, high cholesterol can cause high blood pressure because it makes the heart work too hard.

High cholesterol can be inherited. Familial hypercholesterolemia is when you have inherited a mutated gene that doesn't allow your body to break down or absorb the LDL (bad) cholesterol correctly. Almost ten percent of early-onset heart disease cases are found to have inherited this mutated gene. If you are diagnosed with Familial hypercholesterolemia, your doctor will likely prescribe medication to help reduce your cholesterol levels, recommend a healthy diet and exercise regimen, and do regular blood tests to check your cholesterol levels. There is no cure for Familial hypercholesterolemia, but you can still live an active, healthy life.

Anyone can have high cholesterol—children, slender people, and young adults. It is not just an overweight or elderly person's disease, so when you go to the doctor for yourself or take your child(ren) for their yearly exam, ask them to check your cholesterol.

After researching high cholesterol, I had so many questions about my test results and diagnoses. If my diet or lifestyle caused high cholesterol, then why didn't it present itself in the blood test for the life insurance policy? Would it also have presented itself in that blood test if it was hereditary?

$$6$$

Chapter 6

Slowly, I stop working correctly. I am unsure what to do anymore. Should I use it for energy or expel it from the body? In the meantime, your numbers are increasing by one hundred, one hundred and fifty...you may drink a little more, but that doesn't make you think anything is wrong because you have been working outside, and it is hot! Two hundred....drinking more and going to the bathroom more is nothing out of the ordinary because if you drink more, you go to the toilet more.... Most of the symptoms you experience are asymptomatic, especially in the early stages. Sssshhhh, the longer I am undetected, the more damage I can cause to your organs and your other systems. Silently, I can take your life from within!

Count your blessings if you are one of the lucky ones and get diagnosed before the unimaginable happens!

Type 2 Diabetes is on the rise, not only in America but across the globe. In 2021, the World Health Organization claims that it killed more than 6.7 million people, and it is a pandemic of epic proportions! Diabetes ranks among the top ten causes of death worldwide. Over 550 million people have diabetes worldwide, and they expect that number to be well over 750 million people by the year 2045! 1 in 3 Americans is prediabetic, and three-quarters of them don't even know it! When you are considered prediabetic, it means your blood sugar levels are higher than usual but not high enough to be considered diabetic. Even those who are deemed prediabetic have an increased risk of stroke and cardiovascular issues.

There are two types of diabetes, known as Type 1 and Type 2. Type 1 can occur at any time in life and is likely triggered by an autoimmune response attacking its own body. Type 1 diabetics must take insulin daily to survive because their bodies have stopped making insulin. Currently, there is no cure for Type 1, and medical professionals don't know how to prevent it from occurring. Type 2 can happen anytime during your life, but lifestyle habits often trigger it and can develop gradually. Type 2 is when your body doesn't use the insulin that it produces appropriately, causing your blood sugar to be erratic. Unlike Type 1, Type 2 diabetes can be _delayed_, _reversed_, or even _prevented_ by having good healthy eating habits and regular exercise.

There are several tests your doctor can do to test your blood sugar (glucose) levels. The most common are A1C and fasting blood sugar tests. The A1C, also known as the glycated hemoglobin test, will check how much sugar is attached to your red blood cells, telling them where you fall on the chart below. The fasting blood sugar test, also known as fasting plasma glucose test, shows how much sugar is in your blood. After you eat or drink, your body breaks down the carbohydrates into sugar for energy. If your body functions correctly, insulin and sugar will decrease as it uses it up. If it is not processing insulin correctly or not making enough, you will have too much sugar in your blood, and your fasting blood sugar test will reflect this.

A1C Chart Used for Reference	
Normal	Below 5.7%
Prediabetes	5.7% to 6.4%
Diabetes	6.5% and above

Studies have shown that genetic predisposition, lifestyle choices, habits, and advanced technology are the driving factors in the increased cases of Type 2 diabetes. The new electric versions of bicycles, scooters, and skateboards are fun and exciting but allow us to sit back and relax and not exercise as much. Other lifestyle changes have also affected the population in general – children are discouraged from walking or riding their bikes to school; Schools have drastically reduced or, in some cases, eliminated physical education programs. Television, smartphones, movie watching, video games, and internet surfing have all encouraged the population to be physically inactive.

As sedimentary lifestyles become increasingly common and diets high in fast food, junk food, and high calories prevail, the cases of Type 2 diabetes will steadily increase. Regrettably, this trend is not only limited to adults; They also expect a parallel increase in diagnoses among children and teenagers.

7

Chapter 7

When people hear the word "pandemic," they automatically think of COVID-19 and the year 2020. Rarely does one think about the global rise in chronic diseases such as high blood pressure, high cholesterol, and diabetes, which are no longer limited to adults. This pandemic will far outstretch the reach that COVID-19 had on the world. The studies I've read were alarming, and I am remiss not to share these findings with you.

Alarmingly, these conditions are increasingly affecting children and adolescents. The prevalence of these non-communicable diseases (NCDs) in young people is a growing public health crisis driven by shifts in lifestyle factors such as diet, physical inactivity, and the pervasive availability of unhealthy food options.

High Blood Pressure in Children

Hypertension, once considered a disease of middle-aged and older adults, is now being detected in younger populations. A combination of poor diet, obesity, and sedentary lifestyles has contributed to the rising number of children with high blood pressure. According to research published by the American Heart Association, **obesity is a significant**

risk factor, with studies showing that obese children are four times more likely to develop hypertension than their normal-weight peers. Early intervention is crucial to prevent the long-term consequences of untreated high blood pressure.

Cholesterol in Children

The rising trend of high cholesterol levels in children is concerning and is frequently associated with diets rich in saturated fats and processed foods, essentially due to excessive consumption of fast food and frequent dining out. Children with elevated cholesterol levels face an increased risk of developing atherosclerosis, where the arteries become clogged, leading to cardiovascular diseases sooner in life rather than later. The Centers for Disease Control and Prevention (CDC) report that about 7% of U.S. children and adolescents aged 6–19 years have high total cholesterol levels. Compared to two decades ago, this number has declined. The reduction, in part, can be attributed to public initiatives promoting healthy eating, exercise, and improved screening.

Although the numbers are declining, there is still a lot of work to do to decrease the percentage of children who spend their young and possibly adult lives fighting this severe condition.

Diabetes in Youth

The surge in **childhood obesity** has also fueled an increase in type 2 diabetes, which was once rare among children. This condition, which impairs the body's ability to process blood sugar, is now diagnosed in young people at alarming rates. The American Diabetes Association has pointed out that type 2 diabetes in children is closely associated with obesity and family history of the disease.

Family history is a significant factor in childhood type 2 diabetes. Studies from the American Diabetes Association have shown that having a parent or sibling with Type 2 diabetes increases the risk dramatically.

A substantial number of children diagnosed with type 2 diabetes have a familial connection to the disease.

A recent study by the Centers for Disease Control and Prevention (CDC) indicates that obesity contributes to up to 80% of diabetes diagnoses in children. Obesity is closely associated with insulin resistance, a significant factor in the development of type 2 diabetes in children.

Change Needs to Happen

The modern lifestyle, marked by increased screen time, reduced physical activity, and changes in recreational habits, plays a crucial role in the rising rates of high blood pressure, cholesterol, and diabetes in children. According to a report from the World Health Organization (WHO), children today spend an **alarming** amount of time on sedentary activities, such as watching television, playing video games, and using smartphones, leading to decreased physical activity levels. This modern lifestyle is detrimental to our children, and we should want to change it!

Change should start at home, with parents leading by example. This will benefit your health and well-being while having a significant physical and mental impact on your children.

Research has consistently demonstrated that engaging in physical activities with your children boosts their mental and physical health and fortifies familial ties. Participating in games, walks, swimming, or sports with your children can help alleviate anxiety, depression, and issues with mood regulation. This benefit is often linked to less idle time, which allows children to concentrate on positive activities. On the other hand, excessive screen and television time can expose children to negative influences that they may tend to imitate.

Outside Free Play

Outside "free play" is another positive activity for children with many benefits, such as physical, emotional, and cognitive development.

Outdoor free play also encourages children to be physically active, which is vital to healthy growth. Running, climbing, and jumping develop gross motor skills, improve balance and coordination, and strengthen muscles and bones. Plus, the natural terrain presents diverse challenges, allowing children to use their muscles for enhanced agility and flexibility. Additionally, exposure to sunlight helps the body produce vitamin D, essential for bone development and a robust immune system.

As my children grew up, we implemented rules that promoted healthy physical habits. For example, watching television or playing video games was not allowed if they wanted a break before starting homework after school. However, they were free to play outside, enjoying activities like fort-building, swimming, biking, skating, or any other pastime they chose.

Before implementing the changes mentioned above, my children had the freedom to watch television or play video games. However, I noticed this led to numerous meltdowns, arguments, and overall stress for the entire family. Recognizing it was unhealthy, I made some adjustments, resulting in nothing but positive outcomes. The frequency of meltdowns and arguments significantly decreased, and the children began engaging in their homework without prompting.

American Academy of Pediatrics study found that outdoor play reduces stress, has a calming effect, and helps children cope with challenges. I believe this was why we saw fewer meltdowns and arguments once we started enforcing the rule to play outside.

Family Gardening

Dietary habits are another aspect of modern family life that requires substantial alteration. The convenience of fast food, driven by the hectic pace of most people's lives, has developed into a detrimental habit posing severe health risks to both children and adults. Even small changes can create a significant impact; all it requires is the willingness to make those changes.

Family gardening offers immense benefits, giving children a wealth of physical, emotional, educational, and social rewards. It provides a perfect setting for family bonding and initiating conversations while tending to the garden. Engaging in this hands-on activity helps children develop essential life skills, fosters a deeper connection with nature, boosts mental and physical well-being, and instills a sense of responsibility. Beyond mere planting, family gardening is an excellent means to educate children about nature, accountability, and patience. They learn through tasks such as watering, weeding, and harvesting by being involved from the beginning by selecting plants and participating in the entire gardening process.

You can also make gardening fun by adding decorations or labeling plants with colorful markers. Creating small tasks for each family member ensures everyone can contribute and enjoy the process.

You don't have to start large; you can start small with container gardening, which is a great way to begin and expand later. It's beneficial to grow produce your children enjoy eating, as this will pique their interest in gardening. Familiar favorites include strawberries, carrots, green beans, spinach, and frequently used herbs.

Over the years, we've creatively repurposed various items for our garden. An old wagon, several bed frames, and used two-by-sixes left over from construction projects are just a few examples. It became a delightful family project to paint them, fill them with soil, and watch our garden flourish.

Family gardening is feasible and enjoyable, regardless of where you reside. Techniques such as container gardening, vertical gardening, and raised beds enable cultivating various plants, even in limited spaces. From a handful of herb pots on a windowsill to an expansive vertical garden on a balcony, the advantages of gardening as a family are substantial, fostering healthy habits in any sized space.

Psychological and Social Impact

Obesity, being a significant risk factor for these diseases, can also go beyond the physical aspects. Children who suffer from obesity have a higher chance of being bullied at school; they often experience low self-esteem and social isolation, which can negatively impact their mental health. Research published in the *Journal of Pediatric Psychology* suggests that children with obesity or chronic conditions may experience anxiety, depression, and even behavioral problems due to the stigma associated with their weight or illness.

The encouraging news is that many of these issues can be prevented (except for hereditary factors) or delayed if families take proactive steps early in a child's life. Establishing good habits when children are young and nurturing them throughout their childhood is crucial.

Involvement at local, state, or federal levels is critical to raising awareness about the magnitude of this issue. The increasing prevalence of these burdens in children necessitates urgent policy and healthcare interventions. Homes and schools are the pivotal arenas in this escalating pandemic! Advocating for healthier school meal programs and increased physical activity during the school day can make a significant difference. Initiating the day with exercises like yoga or a group walk around the campus can be beneficial!

Likewise, reducing the consumption of sugary drinks and snacks in schools can have a substantial impact, but this must be mirrored in the home setting. We must abandon the "do as I say, not as I do" attitude and embrace a "lead by example" approach. This approach is vital in altering our mindset and that of our children.

Moreover, public health initiatives must amplify their efforts to raise awareness about the dangers of inadequate nutrition and lack of exercise in children, targeting both parents and their children. Early intervention via family physicians and making parents responsible for fostering healthy eating practices, encouraging regular physical activity, and prioritizing overall well-being is crucial to reversing the growing incidence of chronic illnesses in children.

The Future of Our Children

The future of our children is in our hands. As parents, we can shape that future with a few simple changes in our own lives. By making these changes, our children and grandchildren will mimic our behaviors, thus giving them a better chance at a long and healthy life.

Furthermore, the trend could be significantly reduced if schools, families, neighbors, and local restaurants collaborate to promote healthier lifestyles for children. By courageously addressing these issues, society can help prevent the next generation of children from suffering the long-term consequences of chronic diseases. I have faith that we can do it!

8

Chapter 8

One year and nine months have passed since that significant day in January. It was a day that altered the course of my life. I could have accepted my diagnosis and taken the endless medications my doctor wanted to prescribe, and that would have been the end of it.

Believe me, I wanted to blame it all on post-menopause, but I knew deep down that it was not the only factor that landed me in my doctor's office. So, I did some soul-searching and decided to make some lifestyle changes.

Initially, I consulted with my doctor to determine which medications were essential and which were optional. She concluded that blood pressure medication was necessary and that I should take a low dose of Metformin. Although she strongly recommended cholesterol and insulin treatments, I declined both.

We talked about further measures I should take in addition to medication to reduce my high levels. The doctor suggested changing my diet, incorporating an exercise regimen, and prescribing some vitamins to tackle my other deficiencies.

With the doctor's recommendation, I agreed that I would start a ketogenic diet. This diet, high in fats and low in carbohydrates, induces a metabolic state known as ketosis. During ketosis, the body becomes adept at using fat for energy rather than carbohydrates.

Usually, the body derives energy from carbohydrates, which are broken down into sugars that enter the bloodstream. On a ketogenic diet, the body is deprived of carbohydrates, leading it to burn fat for energy instead. This process produces molecules called ketones, which result from the breakdown of fat.

Next, she emphasized the importance of incorporating exercise into my daily routine. She suggested beginning with light weightlifting and walking. She stressed that maintaining muscle mass becomes increasingly challenging as one ages, making exercise crucial.

Lastly, I need to consume 100 grams or more of protein daily.

She assured me if I took the medication and implemented the new diet and exercise, my numbers would come down.

9

Chapter 9

Determined to succeed, I ordered a keto recipe book and researched the keto diet as soon as I got home.

Adopting the keto diet required a significant shift in mindset. For my entire life, the term 'diet' has been synonymous with low fat and calories. However, the keto diet stands in stark contrast to this concept. Initially, the high fat and calorie content of the recipes was sickening. I had to learn to ignore these numbers and trust my doctor's expertise.

With my doctor's and husband's encouragement, I implemented the changes and started to see results. I was losing weight, and by the fourth month, I had lost almost fifty pounds, and all my numbers were declining. Exciting!

The initial excitement quickly faded; by the fifth month, I was gaining nearly five pounds each week, a development that was quite disheartening and led to emotional distress. However, my doctor reassured me that this is a regular occurrence. She explained that my body had reached a plateau but emphasized that I would resume losing weight soon and encouraged me not to lose hope. I continued on the same plan, but by the end of month six, I was still gaining weight and feeling defeated. My doctor remained hopeful and wanted me to continue with the same plan.

That evening, I started thinking back to when I was pregnant with my second child. To keep the baby's weight down so I could have a VBAC (vaginal birth after cesarean), my doctor put me on a diet and exercise regimen. The diet was low in fat, calories, and sugar, and I had to incorporate high-intensity aerobics at least three times a week. I switched to this diet and incorporated aerobics into my exercise routine without consulting a doctor.

The news was positive at my next doctor's appointment: I had lost weight, and my numbers continued to decrease! Win! I informed my doctor of the changes in my diet and exercise regimen I had made. Although she looked at me skeptically, she agreed I should continue on this path because my numbers positively changed.

Over the next several months, I continued with the new diet and exercise regimen, and I continued to lose weight. My numbers, although slowly, continued to decline as well. I was feeling excellent!

Chapter 10

While post-menopause has played a role in my diagnosis, it was not the sole factor. With that in mind, I researched menopause and menopause studies to understand its impact on women's health and diagnoses later in life.

Research has found Menopause and visceral adipose tissue (VAT - fat a woman gains around her midsection) are strongly connected to Type 2 diabetes, high cholesterol, and high blood pressure. They also found that the greater the accumulation of VAT, the more metabolic dysfunction.

I gain the majority of my weight in my midsection.

Menopause significantly reduces estrogen levels, affecting where a woman's body accumulates weight. During pre-menopause, weight gain may occur in various body parts. However, as women transition to post-menopause, some may begin to experience weight gain in their midsection, a shift that can be potentially life-threatening.

A study published in 2021 in the journal *Menopause* confirmed the risk of VAT and its effects on a woman's health, especially in post-menopause.

Research has also established that VAT is also a risk factor for insulin resistance, which can lead to type 2 diabetes. A recent study published in *The Journal of Clinical Endocrinology & Metabolism* confirmed this.

VAT contributes to insulin resistance and plays a role in lipid metabolism alongside estrogen. Estrogen is crucial in lipid metabolism, helping women maintain higher levels of HDL ("good" cholesterol) and lower levels of LDL ("bad" cholesterol) throughout their lives. However, as women approach pre-menopause and estrogen levels decline, the protective effects that have kept cholesterol levels balanced begin to diminish. Additionally, studies have shown that VAT secretes inflammatory cytokines and adipokines, contributing to arterial stiffening and plaque buildup. This process elevates in postmenopausal women. This combination is especially detrimental to women, which is why heart disease is the leading cause of death among women. In the United States, 44%, or over 60 million women, are living with some form of heart disease.

In addition to VAT accumulation, insulin resistance, decreased estrogen levels, and high blood pressure in menopausal women are also linked to visceral adipose tissue (VAT). High blood pressure is due to VAT's role in promoting inflammation, insulin resistance, and plaque buildup, which are likely to contribute to increased blood pressure in women during Menopause. A study conducted by *Hypertension* found that VAT influenced significantly higher blood pressure than a woman's BMI (body mass index).

In summary, the reduction of estrogen initiates the accumulation of VAT in a woman's body. This VAT then begins to produce inflammatory substances, triggering the onset of insulin resistance. Furthermore, the combination of decreased estrogen and increased VAT undermines lipid metabolism protection, permitting plaque buildup in the arteries, which results in high blood pressure. These issues have a significant impact on a woman's health, increasing her risk for heart disease.

There are things that we as women can do to combat these health issues, and preventive measures could save your life.

Changing your diet is one of the most significant things you can do. A fiber-rich diet, lean proteins, good fats, and whole grains can help limit weight gain. Although this is the recommended diet, we all are different, and our bodies will react differently. I recommend consulting with your doctor and making a plan but remain flexible. Since I knew my body better and had an experience with a diet that worked, making that change kept me on a path to losing weight.

Regular exercise is essential for boosting a slow metabolism and managing or reducing VAT fat. It also aids in preserving muscle mass and enhancing insulin regulation. Alongside exercise, ensure your diet is rich in protein, supporting muscle maintenance. If you notice your weight plateauing, be prepared to adjust your exercise regimen accordingly.

I began with light weightlifting, which I soon found monotonous, so I explored different exercise methods. My routine now includes indoor bouldering, stationary cycling, yoga, aerobics, and light weightlifting. Indoor bouldering is particularly fulfilling for me; it's a comprehensive workout that's both challenging and engaging, significantly since the sections @TheBlokClimbing are updated weekly.

Embrace new experiences to maintain a proactive approach to your health!

11

Chapter 11

Where am I now? Currently, my health metrics have shown significant improvement. The numbers were encouraging at my latest doctor's appointment, with nearly all moving from the "red" zone. I'm pleased with these results! It's clear that my efforts yield benefits, yet I acknowledge there's more to do. I understand the importance of persisting with my routines to maintain this healthier trajectory.

I aim to share my statistics with you to inspire you to make changes that enhance your quality of life. Please consider adjusting your lifestyle before receiving devastating news and before any damage becomes irreversible.

Title	Normal Ranges	Beginning	Now
Weight	108-136	255	143
Fat Mass	3.8 – 8.6	13.5	9.6
BMI	18.5 – 24.0	31.3	26.6
Skeletal Muscle Mass	34.4 – 48.0	43.54	43.15
VAT	0 – 1.2	3.41	1.71
Waist Circumference	< 31"	42"	36"
Glucose	65 - 99	243	145
Vitamin D	50 - 100	34.9	55
A1C	<5.7	11.2	7.2
Cholesterol	<200	299	276
Triglycerides	<150	451	205
HDL	0.00 – 4.44	6.23	4.10
Non-HDL	<130	251	140
LDL Cholesterol	<130	**	163
Blood Pressure	120/80	171/106	114/66

** unable to calculate because triglycerides were over 400

12

REFERENCES

4. "Menopause, visceral fat, and metabolic syndrome in women" - Journal of Clinical Endocrinology & Metabolism (2020). - Bing. (n.d.). Bing. https://www.bing.com/videos/search?q=4.+%22Menopause%2c+visceral+fat%2c+and+metabolic+syndrome+in+women%22+-+Journal+of+Clinical+Endocrinology+%26+Metabolism+(2020).&qpvt=4.+%22Menopause%2c+visceral+fat%2c+and+metabolic+syndrome+in+women%22+-+Journal+of+Clinical+Endocrinology+%26+Metabolism+(2020).&FORM=VDRE

14 Journal of Pediatric Psychology. "Mental Health Outcomes in Children with Chronic Diseases." 2019. - Bing. (n.d.). Bing. https://www.bing.com/videos/search?q=14+Journal+of+Pediatric+Psychology.+%22Mental+Health+Outcomes+in+Children+with+Chronic+Diseases.%22+2019.&qpvt=14+Journal+of+Pediatric+Psychology.+%22Mental+Health+Outcomes+in+Children+with+Chronic+Diseases.%22+2019.&FORM=VDRE

2023 ESH Hypertension Guideline Update: Bringing us Closer Together across the pond - American College of Cardiology. (2024, February 5). American College of Cardiology. https://www.acc.org/latest-in-cardiology/articles/2024/02/05/11/43/2023-esh-hypertension-guideline-update

American Heart Association Understanding Blood Pressure Readings - Bing. (n.d.). Bing. https://www.bing.com/search?pglt=43&q=american+heart+association+understanding+blood+pressure+readings&cvid=9f45a80a7d7b47cea710bb44eea0dec3&gs_lcrp=EgZjaHJvbWUyBggAEEUYOdIBCTEzODY3ajBqMagCCLACAQ&FORM=ANNTA1&PC=U531

Desai, A. N. (2020). High blood pressure. *JAMA*, 324(12), 1254. https://doi.org/10.1001/jama.2020.11289

Diets improve but remain poor for most U.S. children. (2020, April 14). National Institutes of Health (NIH). https://www.nih.gov/news-events/nih-research-matters/diets-improve-remain-poor-most-us-children

ElSayed, N. A., Aleppo, G., Aroda, V. R., Bannuru, R. R., Brown, F. M., Bruemmer, D., Collins, B. S., Hilliard, M. E., Isaacs, D., Johnson, E. L., Kahan, S., Khunti, K., Leon, J., Lyons, S. K., Perry, M. L., Prahalad, P., Pratley, R. E., Seley, J. J., Stanton, R. C., & Gabbay, R. A. (2022). 14. Children and Adolescents: Standards of Care in Diabetes—2023. *Diabetes Care*, 46(Supplement_1), S230–S253. https://doi.org/10.2337/dc23-s014

High blood pressure facts. (2024a, May 15). High Blood Pressure. https://www.cdc.gov/high-blood-pressure/data-research/facts-stats/index.html

High blood pressure facts. (2024b, May 15). High Blood Pressure. https://www.cdc.gov/high-blood-pressure/data-research/facts-stats/index.html

High cholesterol facts. (2024, May 15). Cholesterol. https://www.cdc.gov/cholesterol/data-research/facts-stats/?CDC_AAref_Val=https://www.cdc.gov/cholesterol/facts.htm

Information note on COVID-19 and NCDs. (n.d.). https://www.who.int/publications/m/item/covid-19-and-ncds

James, P. A., Oparil, S., Carter, B. L., Cushman, W. C., Dennison-Himmelfarb, C., Handler, J., Lackland, D. T., LeFevre, M. L., MacKenzie, T. D., Ogedegbe, O., Smith, S. C., Svetkey, L. P., Taler, S. J., Townsend,

R. R., Wright, J. T., Narva, A. S., & Ortiz, E. (2013). 2014 Evidence-Based Guideline for the Management of High Blood Pressure in Adults. *JAMA*, *311*(5), 507. https://doi.org/10.1001/jama.2013.284427

Journal of Hypertension (2020): "Hypertension and Epistaxis: Rare or Exacerbated?" - Bing. (n.d.). Bing. https://www.bing.com/videos/search?q=Journal+of+Hypertension+(2020)%3a+%22Hypertension+and+Epistaxis%3a+Rare+or+Exacerbated%3f%22&qpvt=Journal+of+Hypertension+(2020)%3a+%22Hypertension+and+Epistaxis%3a+Rare+or+Exacerbated%3f%22&FORM=VDRE

Khoury, N., Martínez, M. Á., Garcidueñas-Fimbres, T. E., Pastor-Villaescusa, B., Leis, R., De Las Heras-Delgado, S., Miguel-Berges, M. L., Navas-Carretero, S., Portoles, O., Pérez-Vega, K. A., Jurado-Castro, J. M., Vázquez-Cobela, R., Mimbrero, G., Horno, R. A., Martínez, J. A., Flores-Rojas, K., Picáns-Leis, R., Luque, V., Moreno, L. A., . . . Babio, N. (2024). Ultra-processed food consumption and cardiometabolic risk factors in children. *JAMA Network Open*, 7(5), e2411852. https://doi.org/10.1001/jamanetworkopen.2024.11852

Management-Screening, Diagnosis and Treatment (MND). (2016, April 21). *Global report on diabetes.* https://www.who.int/publications/i/item/9789241565257

Management-Screening, Diagnosis and Treatment (MND). (2019, April 21). *Classification of diabetes mellitus.* https://www.who.int/publications/i/item/classification-of-diabetes-mellitus

Menopause. (n.d.). https://journals.lww.com/menopausejournal

Nguyen, D., Kit, B., Carroll, M., U.S. DEPARTMENT OF HEALTH AND HUMAN SERVICES, Centers for Disease Control and Prevention, & National Center for Health Statistics. (2015). Abnormal cholesterol among children and adolescents in the United States, 2011–2014. In *NCHS Data Brief* (No. 228). https://www.cdc.gov/nchs/data/databriefs/db228.pdf

Non-communicable Diseases, Rehabilitation and Disability

(NCD). (2013, November 14). *Global action plan for the prevention and control of non-communicable diseases 2013-2020.* https://www.who.int/publications/i/item/9789241506236

Powell-Wiley, T. M., Poirier, P., Burke, L. E., Després, J., Gordon-Larsen, P., Lavie, C. J., Lear, S. A., Ndumele, C. E., Neeland, I. J., Sanders, P., & St-Onge, M. (2021). Obesity and Cardiovascular Disease: A scientific statement from the American Heart Association. *Circulation, 143*(21). https://doi.org/10.1161/cir.0000000000000973

Touyz, R. M. (2022). Hypertension 2022 Update: Focusing on the future. *Hypertension, 79*(8), 1559–1562. https://doi.org/10.1161/hypertensionaha.122.19564

Type 2 diabetes in children - Symptoms and causes - Mayo Clinic. (2023, November 18). Mayo Clinic. https://www.mayoclinic.org/diseases-conditions/type-2-diabetes-in-children/symptoms-causes/syc-20355318

World Health Organization: WHO & World Health Organization: WHO. (2023, April 5). *Diabetes.* https://www.who.int/news-room/fact-sheets/detail/diabetes

Steele, M. M., Graves, M. M., Roberts, M. C., & Steele, R. G. (2006). Examining the Influence of the Journal of Pediatric Psychology: An Empirical Approach. Journal of Pediatric Psychology. https://doi.org/10.1093/jpepsy/jsj111

www.ingramcontent.com/pod-product-compliance
Lightning Source LLC
Chambersburg PA
CBHW061535250726
48657CB00005B/2242